Defeat Hypertension Unlock Longevity

The Ultimate Guide to Manage High Blood Pressure, Prevent Related Chronic Diseases and Achieve Healthy Long Life

Prateek Asthana

Copyright © 2024 Prateek Asthana
All rights reserved. No part of this publication may be reproduced, distributed or transmitted in any form or by any means including photocopying, recording or other mechanical, electrical methods without the prior written permission of the publisher.

About the Author

Prateek Asthana has been into fitness industry by passion for over 15+ years; here are some of his key achievements:
- ✓ Author of the bestseller books 'Add Fitness to Lifestyle' and 'Eat Mindfully Cheat Wisely'
- ✓ Certified Fitness Trainer (International Sports Science Association)
- ✓ Certified in Sports Nutrition (International Sports Science Association)
- ✓ Certified Black Belt Dan-I in Taekwondo (from Orient Combat Arts in association with World Taekwondo Federation, Kukkiwon, Korea)
- ✓ Certified Life Coach
- ✓ Ex-Fitness Consultant in Healthifyme
- ✓ Gold medalist in the Open Taekwondo Corporate Championship held at District Level in Pune under the 66-75Kg Weight Category in 2016
- ✓ Intermediate Level in Boxing & Kickboxing
- ✓ Competed in National and International Half Marathons
- ✓ Certified in First Aid and CPR

and he loves to play outdoor sports like squash, badminton and cricket.

He started his fitness journey over 15 years back with resistance training. Prateek has also participated in half marathons from 2015-2018, including one international marathon. He joined martial arts classes in mid-2016 and achieved black belt in 2019 end. In parallel, he also learnt boxing and kickboxing. With years of experience in fitness, he decided to take it to the next level by doing fitness training and sports nutrition certifications, after which he worked as a fitness consultant at HealthifyMe for a short duration.

By education, he is an IT professional and he respects his primary job and loves learning new things in the fitness industry. Prateek stays in Pune (India) and has recently joined calisthenics classes to learn and master a new skill.

You can connect with him on his personal account:
Instagram (prateek_asthana_)
Facebook (www.facebook.com/prateek.asthana.3)

Contents

Chapter 1: High Blood Pressure- A Silent Killer 6

Chapter 2: Blood Pressure Measurement and Categories 9

Chapter 3: Blood Circulation and Pressure Complications . 14

Chapter 4: Borderline BP Reading' Importance 16

Chapter 5: The Gray Zone Around Hypertension Medication 18

Chapter 6: Key Factors to Obtain Accurate Blood Pressure Readings 21

Chapter 7: How to Know Whether Your Blood Pressure Monitor at Home is Accurate? 24

Chapter 8: High Blood Pressure Leading to Organ Damage 26

    The Heart: Most Vulnerable Organ 27

    Stroke: Danger to the Brain 31

    Eyes: Most Sensitive Organ 33

    Sex Organs: Care For Your Desires 37

    Kidney Failure: Normal Urine is a Bliss 38

Chapter 9: Factors affecting Blood Pressure 41

Chapter 10: Medications & Prescriptions That Can Cause High Blood Pressure 50

Chapter 11: Benefits, Risks and Side-effects of BP Medications 57

Chapter 12: When Do You Actually Need Medicine for High Blood Pressure? 61

Chapter 13: Combination Therapy for Managing High BP .. 64

    Challenges Associated with Combination Therapy 67

Strategies to Overcome the Challenges of Combination Therapy 68

Chapter 14: Avoid Interference with Other Medicines 71

Chapter 15: Follow-Up Questions to Ask Your Healthcare Professional 73

Chapter 16: What if Your Left and Right Sides Have Different BP Readings 77

Chapter 17: Workouts for High Blood Pressure 79

   Other Factors During Workout 85

Chapter 18: Nutrition for High Blood Pressure 88

   Mediterranean Diet 90

Chapter 19: Factors that might help you in Quick Fixes for Extreme Cases 94

Chapter 20: Effects of Caffeine on High Blood Pressure 99

Chapter 21: Other Helpful Factors 102

Chapter 21: Closure 106

Chapter 1: High Blood Pressure- A Silent Killer

Your blood pressure reading is crucial since failing to check that could be fatal. High blood pressure is referred to as the "silent killer," and it is a very reliable indicator of your internal health. It's "silent" because, generally speaking, you never feel your blood pressure being dangerously high. Most individuals really cannot tell when their blood pressure is elevated; a few fortunate people may notice symptoms like swollen ankles, headaches, dizziness, or blurred vision. Prolonged high blood pressure steals life and energy by slowly depriving your cells and tissues of blood flow and seriously harming your key organs.

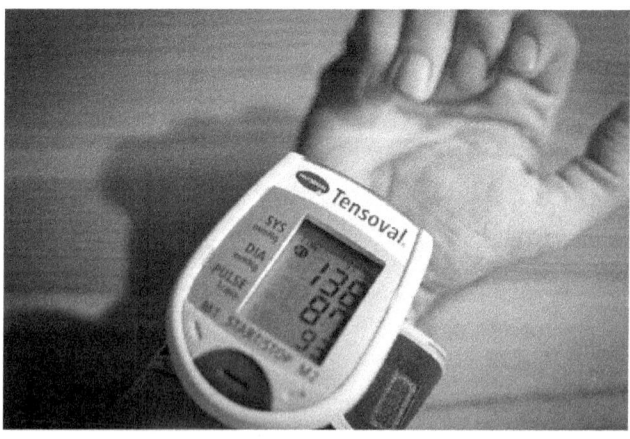

The two figures in a blood pressure reading provide us with a wealth of information on the condition of your internal organs, particularly in relation to the heart and arteries' resilience. Cardiovascular disease, which is the main cause of death for people worldwide, is brought on by high blood pressure.

The heart, brain, and kidneys are the body components most in need of a steady blood flow, and they suffer greatly from hypertension. This implies that even a small increase in blood pressure can strangle these organs due to limited blood flow, increasing your risk of heart attack, stroke, and chronic renal disease, which can require dialysis. Literally, high blood pressure can be fatal. Research demonstrates that if you are diagnosed with hypertension due to very high numbers, your health and lifespan are clearly at risk.

The Definition of High Blood Pressure

When the heart has to work harder than usual to pump blood through your arteries and into your tissues and organs, you have high blood pressure, often known as hypertension, HTN, or HBP. They will diagnose you with "high blood pressure" if the force of your blood pressing against the walls of your blood vessels is too high. This precarious scenario is the result of a plethora of contributing factors and occurrences. The earlier you get to know about it, the sooner we can consult the doctor and take the required action to control or reverse this medical condition, be it making changes to your lifestyle chances or the taking drugs required to control it.

Chapter 2: Blood Pressure Measurement and Categories

Blood Pressure Measurement

Using a cuff that either manually or electronically reports two forces, we take your blood pressure.
Systolic pressure, the highest figure, is the result of blood pumping from the heart into the arteries.
Diastolic pressure, the lowest value, is produced when the heart relaxes or rests in between heartbeats.

In other words, if your blood pressure is 140/90, the upper number indicates how hard the heart must pump, and the bottom number indicates how much back pressure remains when the heart is relaxed. Excessive pressure, as indicated by either figure, can cause major difficulties and organ damage. For every 20 mm Hg systolic or 10 mm Hg diastolic increase in blood pressure above 120/80 in those 40 to 89 years of age, the chance of dying from a stroke or heart attack doubles!

Since years ago, the permitted range for blood pressure readings has decreased since scientists are increasingly understanding how the excessive pressure damages our organs and vessels. When the patient was an elderly person decades ago, blood pressure readings of 160/90 mm Hg were not considered dangerous. In hindsight, something is not always normal just because it is frequent. These elevated blood pressure values that were deemed "normal" most likely caused numerous avoidable problems. A few decades later, the maximum limit was changed, and 140/90 was established as the standard blood pressure reading. Even that, in our opinion today, is too high. Only blood pressures less than 120/80 are considered normal by the American Heart Association, and excessive blood pressure can now be formally diagnosed at any repeat reading over 119 or 79.

This indicates that because 130/80 or greater is now considered hypertension, nearly half of Americans are now officially diagnosed with high blood pressure. Over 180/120 is referred to as a hypertensive crisis, and anything over 140/90 is considered Stage 2 hypertension.

Blood Pressure Categories

The American Heart Association lists these five blood pressure categories as of 2017. We had a category termed "pre-hypertension" until a few years ago. That was removed by the expert guidelines in 2017, and we now refer to that as "elevated blood pressure."

1. Normal Blood Pressure

Less than 120/80 mm Hg is regarded as being within the normal range for blood pressure measurements. If this is the case with your results, continue with heart-healthy practices such as eating a balanced diet and exercising on a regular basis.

2. Elevated Blood Pressure

A consistently high blood pressure reading falls between 120 and 129 mm Hg at the systolic and less than 80 mm Hg at the diastolic levels. Individuals who have high blood pressure are more likely to develop high blood pressure if they don't take action to manage their condition.

3. Hypertension Stage 1

When blood pressure constantly falls between 80 and 89 mm Hg diastolic or between 130 and 139 systolic, it is referred to as stage 1 hypertension. Depending on your individual or family risks, doctors may recommend lifestyle modifications and blood pressure medication at this stage of high blood pressure, particularly if you have a history of cardiovascular disease, heart attacks, or strokes.

There have been a number of cases where people have even reversed this stage by altering their lifestyle by increasing physical activity and eating a healthy diet even without taking medication.

4. Hypertension Stage 2

When blood pressure continuously varies at 140/90 mm Hg or higher, it is considered hypertension stage 2. Doctors are likely to recommend a mix of blood pressure drugs and lifestyle modifications at this stage of high blood pressure.

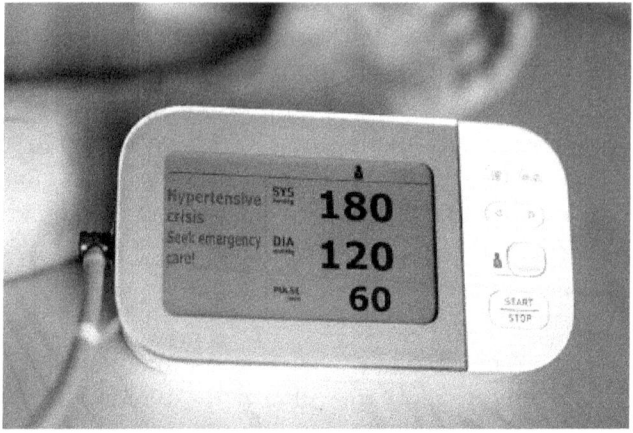

5. Hypertensive Crisis

When high blood pressure reaches this point, immediate medical intervention is needed. In the event that your blood pressure readings unexpectedly rise above 180/120 mm Hg, give yourself five minutes before taking another reading. Get in touch with your healthcare provider right away if your readings are still abnormally high. It is possible that you are having a hypertensive crisis.

Do not wait to see whether your blood pressure lowers on its own if it is higher than 180/120 mm Hg and you are exhibiting symptoms that could indicate organ damage, such as chest pain, shortness of breath, back pain, numbness or weakness, changes in vision, or difficulty speaking. Seek immediate medical attention.

Chapter 3: Blood Circulation and Pressure Complications

For optimal vitality and energy, your tissues and organs require a fresh supply of oxygenated blood every few seconds. Your lungs' air sacs give oxygen to red blood cells that are traveling through the bloodstream with every breath. The circulatory system, which is made up of arteries and capillaries, pumps this oxygenated blood from the lungs throughout your body and back again.

In the event of increased resistance, the flow rate must decrease to sustain pressure, or the pressure must rise to sustain flow. Although there are many variables that might affect resistance, the three most crucial ones are blood viscosity, or how thick and sticky your blood is, vessel radius, and vascular length. Resistance increases with increasing length, increasing viscosity, and decreasing radius. In addition, the pressure in the arteries nearer the heart is higher than in the veins in the limbs. It makes sense that doing this requires a lot of heart muscle strength.

For the duration of your life, the arteries, arterioles, and microscopic capillaries that comprise these blood vessels endure the heaviest portion of this pressure pump with each and every pulse.

Hypertension Complications

Assume you have a garden hose that has a weak point. If you slowly turn on the water spigot, nothing is likely to happen; the same is likely to happen if you increase the pressure. However, that tiny weak point might not hold, and the hose will leak, if you make a knot in it and then turn on the water or abruptly alter the pressure by going from off to full force quickly. An analogous event may transpire within your arteries. The following dangerous consequences of hypertension are brought on by high blood pressure's weakening of the arteries and organs:

- Stroke
- Heart attack
- Congestive heart failure
- Kidney failure
- Sexual dysfunction
- Blindness

Everything relies on your areas of vulnerability and the location of the issue. Fortunately, if we manage or better yet, reverse your high blood pressure, all of these can be avoided.

So, maintaining a normal blood pressure means protecting your heart, brain, kidneys, arteries, eyes, and sex organs in a way.

Chapter 4: Borderline BP Reading' Importance

The American Medical Association, the American Heart Association, and the CDC (Centers for Disease Control and Prevention) released updated in-office guidelines in 2017 regarding the proper way for physicians and dentists to take blood pressure readings. The number of people who receive a hypertension diagnosis will undoubtedly be impacted by these new regulations.
Since a few easy steps may typically reverse hypertension, this is also a great chance to raise awareness and boost up efforts to take therapeutic lifestyle changes seriously in order to prevent future problems.

Moreover, home blood pressure monitoring appears to be an essential first step toward regulating blood pressure and averting consequences, particularly hypertension-mediated organ damage (HMOD). If blood sugar readings from doctor's offices were the only ones we used, just think of how inadequately we could treat diabetes! This also applies to blood pressure. We must witness it in all phases of your existence—the happy and the sad, the relaxed and the anxious, the contented and the agitated.

Patients with 24-hour ambulatory blood pressure monitoring (ABPM) or those who take regular home readings with an automated cuff are able to take more accurate blood pressure readings outside of the office. They appear to be more repeatable than office measurements and, more significantly, they have a stronger correlation with the risk of a heart attack, stroke, or organ damage caused by hypertension.

A true minority of patients—between 10 and 30 percent—have blood pressure that rises solely in the presence of medical personnel. However, 10 to 15 percent of the population suffers from "masked hypertension," a condition in which a person's blood pressure is normal when measured in the office but frequently jumps at home. If home blood pressure monitoring is not used, it is simple for medical professionals to misdiagnose hypertension and lose accuracy.

Chapter 5: The Gray Zone Around Hypertension Medication

There is still a huge gray zone around what constitutes hypertension and when (drug) treatment should begin.

The 2017 American Heart Association guidelines for normal, elevated, hypertension stage 1, hypertension stage 2 and hypertension crises have already been covered. Other companies, though, do not make use of the same architecture.

The 2020 International Society of Hypertension (Global Hypertension Practice Guidelines), does not declare hypertension unless BP is 140/90 or greater. Systolic pressure below 130 and diastolic pressure below 85 is considered normal blood pressure. "High-normal" blood pressure is defined as 130–139 or 85–89. Although, home blood pressure monitoring for this group is highly recommended.

The World Health Organization's 2022 standards, however, changed the assessment guidelines. Their levels vary based on co-morbidities, or any conditions you might have in addition to hypertension. If a person's blood pressure is more than 90 diastolic and 140 systolic, they are diagnosed with hypertension even if they simply have a high reading.

However, if you already have cardiovascular disease, a measurement of more above 130 systolic indicates that you are hypertensive. A diagnosis is also made if you are over 130 and do not currently have cardiovascular disease but are at risk due to diabetes, chronic renal disease, or atherosclerosis in your neck or leg arteries. (Plaque accumulation in artery walls known as atherosclerosis can obstruct blood flow and result in a stroke, heart attack or other problems.)

The U.S. Preventive Service Task Force stated in 2021 that hypertension is characterized as a blood pressure reading of 140/90 mm Hg or more than 130/80 mm Hg. This organization left the decision-making for your specific case to your doctors. It is obvious that there is disagreement among professionals over the precise definition of hypertension. Declaring your diagnosis may also depend on your specific co-morbidities and the professional association to which your physician belongs.

When the terms "maximum acceptable" as opposed to "target reading" are used, patients and their physicians take much more aggressive approach to treatment. Consider the scenario where your blood pressure is 145/92. There isn't much reason for you or your doctor to adjust if your target is 140/90 because you are already within the target range. Adjustments must be done immediately if your maximum allowable reading is 140/90, as both the 145 and the 92 are obviously too high.

Every organization concurs that the risk of HMOD (hypertension-mediated organ damage) is nearly nonexistent at a normal blood pressure of less than 120/80. Obtaining correct readings is crucial. We don't want to misdiagnose hypertensive patients because we took the wrong reading! Nor do we want to overtreat our patients. It is important for patients and their physicians to understand that deviating from the recommended course of action might lead to erroneous rises in blood pressure measurements and possibly an overdiagnosis of a serious illness.

Chapter 6: Key Factors to Obtain Accurate Blood Pressure Readings

Make sure you are motionless and quiet for five minutes before taking your blood pressure. When you are waiting or having your blood pressure taken, you shouldn't be chit-chatting with the office personnel or checking your phone! Just stay still and don't listen in on those intriguing discussions taking place in the doctor's office. These guidelines for taking an accurate blood pressure reading are as follows:

- Clear your bladder before checking your blood pressure.
- Do not smoke, drink or eat for 30 minutes before you measure your blood pressure.
- Again, do not talk or even listen intently to someone while your readings are being taken.
- Do not put your blood pressure cuff over your clothing. It should go on your bare arm.
- Your arm shouldn't be hanging by your side; it should be level with your heart. For at least five minutes, you must recline completely in the chair with your back supported.
- Your legs or ankles cannot be crossed. Straighten your legs and keep your feet on the floor or a stool without dangling.

Impacts of the Above Points on Your BP Reading

- When you eat within 30 minutes of getting your blood pressure checked, it can go up by 4 mm Hg diastolic and 3 mm Hg systolic.
- 12 ounces of coffee can raise blood pressure by 8 mm Hg in the systolic and 6 mm Hg in the diastolic ranges. Smoking raises the diastolic pressure by 4 mm Hg and the systolic pressure by 7 mm Hg.
- Your blood pressure reading may increase by 10 to 40 mm Hg if you place the blood pressure cuff over a shirt or sweater instead than on bare skin.
- A severely full bladder might result in an elevation of 10 to 15 points, which can remain for three hours.
- How many times did you have to "hold it" too long knowing that your doctor would need a urine sample when you got to the office? While it might facilitate the provision of a urine sample, it could lead to an imprecise assessment of blood pressure.
- Talking or even listening carefully might raise blood pressure by 10 to 15 mm Hg. Speaking can have a worse effect on your blood pressure the higher it is in the first place. Some hypertensive people saw a 25–40% increase in blood pressure in just 30 seconds after they started speaking.

- ➢ You can increase your readings by 10 mm Hg if you don't support the arm at heart level and instead let it hang at your side.
- ➢ The act of utilizing your back muscles when seated in a chair without support can result in an additional 5 to 10 mm Hg.
- ➢ When seated, dangling your feet can cause your reading to be off by 5 to 10 mm Hg.
- ➢ When having your blood pressure checked, crossing your legs can cause an increase of 2 to 8 mm Hg.

Any one of these typical errors can easily cause you to receive an inaccurately high blood pressure measurement. If you make two or three errors in a row, you may be placed in a higher risk category. So, pick up these easy tips to assist your doctor in gathering the most correct information for your treatment.

Nevertheless, I advise you to abide by the guidelines as this will help you and your primary care physician become better patients. Additionally, I ask that you refrain from educating your doctor or nurse about the most recent guidelines as our joint objective should be to normalize our blood pressure readings. Treat everyone with kindness!

Chapter 7: How to Know Whether Your Blood Pressure Monitor at Home is Accurate?

For this goal, a streamlined version of the European Society of Hypertension International Protocol has been created, which you and your physician may complete quickly. This can be found in the American Heart Association's Million Hearts PDF.

This is the comparative exam for ten minutes:

- Prior to beginning the readings, make sure you have completed all the prerequisites that we have discussed.
- Take five consecutive measures of your blood pressure using the same arm, no more than 30 seconds apart.
- Using a personal device, take the first two readings.
- Make sure your physician obtains the third reading, ideally using a comparable contemporary electronic device or an antiquated mercury sphygmomanometer.
- On your personal gadget, you take the fourth reading.
- This is the fifth and last reading that your physician takes.
- Examine how the readings from the two cuffs differ from one another.

➢ Over the course of the five measures, blood pressure readings will nearly invariably drop. Up to 10 mm Hg less systolic blood pressure was recorded in the last reading than in the initial one. The comparison is permitted if the difference is 5 mm Hg or less. Repeat the calibration if the discrepancy is more than 5 mm Hg but less than 10 mm Hg. The instrument might not be accurate if the differential is more than 10 mm Hg.

Once a year, carry out this process again.

While there isn't a set standard for how closely the patient's and the doctor's cuff readings should match, this exercise can give you a general idea of how accurate the self-measured blood pressure monitoring device is. You can then take that into account for your own future home measurements.

Chapter 8: High Blood Pressure Leading to Organ Damage

Assume your blood pressure is typically 139/89 and you have stage 1 hypertension. But then due to any mishap, like getting caught in a snowstorm, that made your blood pressure surge abnormally high, and you had to use a shovel to get out of your house. Your blood pressure shot up to 180/100 all of a sudden. This is referred to as a hypertensive urgency, and it needs to be treated quickly in order to try to get it out of danger. In five to ten minutes, it should be retested. Until then, we can continue to closely monitor you if you are symptom-free.

If your blood pressure is 180/100 and you experience difficulties speaking, numbness or weakness, back discomfort, chest pain, or changes in eyesight. If so, you are experiencing a hypertensive crisis and need to get emergency medical attention right once. Abrupt elevation of blood pressure may lead to insufficient blood flow, suffocating the organs with the smallest blood arteries. This implies that the organs most vulnerable are those with the tiniest arteries. By examining the organs that are impacted, we shall examine the possible meanings of each of these symptoms:
- ➢ Heart
- ➢ Kidneys
- ➢ Brain
- ➢ Eyes
- ➢ Sex Organs

The Heart: Most Vulnerable Organ

The heart is the organ most vulnerable to a hypertensive crisis. It is a little perplexing since the surface of the heart has some of the smaller arteries, but it also includes some of the largest blood vessels in the body that leave it and flow to the lungs and limbs. These tiny arteries, known as "coronary arteries," provide the heart muscle with blood and oxygen. The entire heart muscle "south" of the obstruction is in danger if they are strangled or if a blood clot forms inside of them.

Angina

Large portions of the heart's pumping chambers are supplied by the coronary arteries, thus if they are weakened, angina or a heart attack may result. Angina is a transient form of chest pain that does not cause permanent harm, but it is vital to get evaluated since the pain pattern is the same as that of a heart attack. Your healthcare practitioner can determine if you need to stay in the hospital for a few days or if you may be treated and sent home with the use of an ECG or EKG tracking and some blood testing.

Rhythm Disturbances

The heart can rapidly go out of rhythm if the damaged veins are in a region that supplies blood to the pacemaker cells. Shortness of breath, chest pain, and a feeling of an irregular heartbeat or fluttering in the chest are all signs of an out-of-rhythm heart. The bottom two chambers of the heart are referred to as the "ventricles," and the top two chambers as the "atria." If your heartbeats are in time, you will hear the distinctive "lub dub" sound.

Atrial Fibrillation

A targeted heart shock treatment or medication can occasionally reverse or at least control atrial fibrillation, one of the rhythm disorders that can occur during a heart attack. The heart "quivers" on top, causing the pulse to become erratic. A "dub" beat will then sporadically emerge from the bottom chamber. As you lose the excess blood volume from the atrial pumping action, you may experience weakness and shortness of breath.

Ventricular Fibrillation

Ventricular fibrillation, or "v-fib," is a further, much more dangerous consequence. This more severe rhythm irregularity causes "v-fib," which results in abrupt death by stopping the bottom chamber from pumping at all. Within minutes, v-fib can be fatal unless a bystander can do CPR or has access to an automatic defibrillator. By learning how to use a defibrillator and do CPR, we can all benefit our communities.

Rising Cardiovascular Diseases

The prevalence of cardiovascular disease is still rising in spite of all of our efforts in public awareness campaigns and education. While one in three American women dies from a heart attack, one in thirty-one dies from breast cancer, despite the fact that many women fears dying from the disease. Compared to our breasts, our hearts are ten times more vulnerable.

The long-term statistics after a heart attack are alarming. 35% percent of men and 47% percent of women die within the first year after a heart attack.

The general public's knowledge that heart disease is a leading cause of death is dwindling over time. In 2016, more than 66% of individuals surveyed were aware that heart disease was the leading cause of death in the country; however, by 2019, only 44% of them still understood this, presumably as a result of a lack of public health awareness or other unspecified circumstances. There is still a great deal of effort to be done to raise awareness of this dangerous but mostly preventable health issue.

The outlook for our cardiovascular system is likewise not too bright. Many specialists predict that the number of heart attacks and strokes will rise by thirty percent, by the year 2060. This need not take place. If we alter our diet to include more nutrient-dense foods, increase our physical activity, get deep, restorative sleep, and pinpoint and address the underlying causes of our elevated blood pressure and inflammation, we can reverse the trends and prevent the majority, if not all, of these cardiovascular events.

Common Signs and Symptoms

Chest Discomfort
The majority of heart attacks are characterized by pain in the middle of the chest that either persists for a few minutes or briefly disappears before returning. It may experience pain, fullness, squeezing, or uncomfortable pressure.

Body Discomfort
The back, neck, jaw, stomach, and one or both arms may all experience pain or discomfort as symptoms.

Breathlessness
May occur with or without discomfort in the chest.

Additional symptoms could be lightheadedness, nausea, or a chilly sweat.

Gender Differences
It's crucial to understand that women frequently have no chest pain during a heart attack. It is important that we acknowledge gender differences and, in some situations, that we inform our family members and medical professionals of this information.

The most common symptoms of a heart attack in women are:

- Discomfort in the neck, jaw, shoulder, upper back, or upper abdomen (not even pain).
- Breathlessness, also referred to as "getting easily winded."
- One or both arms hurt.
- Vomiting or nausea
- Perspiration or sweating
- Dizziness or lightheadedness
- Unusual exhaustion or fatigue.
- Indigestion
- Heartburn

Stroke: Danger to the Brain

Another target organ in danger of harm from a hypertensive crisis is the brain. There is one big carotid artery on each side of the neck. You may locate your carotid artery and feel your pulse there by feeling for the "Adam's apple" on the front of your neck and sliding over approximately an inch to each side into a tiny hollow. The carotids are the size of a pencil, but with each tiny branching-off point as they descend more into your brain, they get smaller. A strand of hair is around the size of some of the arteries in your brain. The elevated pressure in the carotid can force a small blood clot deeper into these tiny cerebral arteries if it forms there.

The term "stroke" refers to both kinds of "brain attacks." Similar to how different wires service different places on your home's circuit panel, different sections of your brain are in charge of distinct functions.

You may get double or blurry vision if a high-pressure event affects the area of your brain located in the back where vision is processed. Even strange blackout locations in your field of vision, such losing vision in only the right side of both eyes, are possible. You can experience a loss of strength in the muscles that are supplied by the damaged motor cortex. This may cause your face muscles to droop, your arm or leg muscles to weaken or even completely paralyze, or cause your muscles to contract in order to hold back pee or feces. Occasionally, signs of a brain injury are more widespread; the entire brain malfunctions, causing you to lose consciousness or faint. outside. Occasionally, memory problems cause you to forget crucial information, such as the date or even your own name.

Common signs of a stroke

Identify a Stroke using **FAST** principle:

Facial drooping: Is one side of the face numb or does it droop? Request a smile from the person.

A Weak Arm: Is one arm numb or weak? Request that they lift both of their arms. Does one arm sag to the side?

Speech Difficulties: Do they have trouble speaking or understanding others? Request that the subject repeat a brief statement, such as "The sky is blue." Is the phrase rephrased accurately?

Time to visit a doctor: Make sure to visit a doctor and take the person to the hospital right away if they exhibit any of these symptoms, even if they pass. A stroke is not always the cause of abrupt weakness in the arms or face, slurred speech, or memory issues. However, an immediate assessment is necessary since the sooner a stroke is treated, the less severe and long-lasting the symptoms may be.

Eyes: Most Sensitive Organ

The eye is another organ with small blood arteries that could be harmed by a hypertension emergency. The eyes' tiny blood vessels make them incredibly vulnerable, even though they are fundamentally a part of the brain. It's important to keep in mind that retinal hemorrhages caused by high blood pressure may lead to blindness if left untreated. This is why you should seek medical assistance as soon as possible if you see a red curtain suddenly obstructing your field of view.

The white part of the eye, known as the sclera, can break blood arteries, which is a common problem unrelated to blood pressure. Known as "sub-conjunctival hemorrhage," they can result in a frighteningly striking brilliant red pool of blood on the white part of the eyeball. These are typically not very related to blood pressure. It looks a lot like a skin bruise, with the exception that it's on the surface of your eyeball. There is no need for care if there is no discomfort, discharge from the eyes, or alteration in vision.

Still, vision changes like a curtain being pulled over one or both eyes, cobwebs or haze, or a red tint to the vision might result from rupturing a blood vessel on the retina, or the back of the eyeball. If this suddenly happens, call your eye care professional or go to the nearest emergency room. However, because strokes often result in vision and balance impairments, many hospital systems have adopted a more modern approach to teach people about early diagnosis of stroke and the significance of seeking emergency care. Early detection increases your chances of curing a stroke and lessening its long-term effects.
So, instead of just asking us to act FAST, they are pushing us to act FASTER.

Face: Examine whether one side of the face is drooping or number than the other. To make the droop more noticeable, ask the subject to smile.

Arms: Determine whether one arm is more numb or weaker than the other. Request that the person raise both arms, then keep them there for ten counts. A stroke may be indicated if one arm drops or begins to fall.

Stability: While standing, check your stability. People occasionally faint, feel extremely lightheaded, or become unable to stand without support. Loss of coordination, problems walking, and difficulty keeping balance are all potential symptoms of a stroke.

Talking: Look for speech abnormalities, such as slurred or garbled words, incoherent sentences, or an inability to reply correctly. People who are having a stroke could be hard to comprehend or could find it hard to understand other people. Request that the individual repeat a brief statement, such as "The sky is blue."

Eyes: Look for any changes in appearance. These abrupt changes in vision might include double vision, partial vision loss in one or both eyes, and complete vision loss in one eye.

React: See a physician right away if you experience any of these signs. Even if the symptoms disappear, give us a call and try to recall when they started.

A visit to the emergency hospital is required if any of these neurological symptoms appear out of the blue. If your situation meets the criteria, an IV (Intravenous – in a vein) can be used to provide clot-busting medications in order to dissolve the clot that caused your symptoms and restore blood flow to the damaged part of your brain. But this needs to be done as quickly as possible—ideally, no later than sixty minutes after the commencement of symptoms.

We refer to it as the "Golden Hour" because there is a greater probability of reducing the handicap the earlier assistance is received. Stroke continues to be the leading cause of long-term impairment because most are too big or occurred too long ago for the amazing clot-buster medications to be effective.

Remember that you can avoid strokes by learning the appropriate preventive techniques.

Peripheral Artery Disease
Peripheral Artery Disease (PAD) poses a significant risk to the arteries in the legs. The narrowing of arteries in the head, arms, stomach, and legs due to atherosclerosis, which is brought on by high blood pressure, inflammation, and tainted cholesterol can result in decreased blood flow and crippling leg pain or weariness that makes walking impossible. Too little is said about PAD. Skin abnormalities, such as cold skin temperature or fragile, glossy skin on the feet and lower legs, can be symptoms.

Many patients report that their toenails harden and turn yellow, and that they can no longer grow hair on their legs. Wounds that are superficial refuse to heal. The legs appear pasty and pale when lying down, but as you stand up, they take on an unusual reddish-purplish color. Sleep might be disrupted by persistent burning discomfort in the feet. The fact that people with PAD—even those who also have high blood pressure or diabetes—are linked to an increased risk of stroke, heart attack, and leg amputation—three times, six times, and eight times, respectively—makes the condition extremely dangerous. By feeling the pulses in your feet, taking your leg blood pressure and comparing it to your arm blood pressure, or scheduling a leg ultrasound, your doctor can assist ascertain whether you have peripheral arterial disease (PAD).

Sex Organs: Care For Your Desires

The sex organs are one organ that is not usually impacted by acute hypertension, but they are also one that is not talked about enough when chronic hypertension is present. Yes, elevated blood pressure does have an impact on the genitalia. Your romantic life may suffer greatly if high blood pressure reduces the blood flow to your sex organs. These small arteries are also destroyed by low blood pressure. Engorgement and swelling during sexual desire should be the result of increased blood flow in the clitoris or penis.

The blood vessels supplying the clitoris and penis may narrow due to atherosclerotic vascular disease, reducing blood flow and possibly resulting in sexual dysfunction. Men with erectile dysfunction (ED), which is defined as the inability to achieve or maintain an erection long enough to complete sexual activity, may encounter problems in this system.

When a man asks to be prescribed Viagra®, he should be thoroughly evaluated for hypertensive vascular disease. In my opinion, a person's penis is a reliable sign of both general health and any malfunction.

Naturally, women and girls are also impacted. This can lead to decreased clitoral blood flow in women and, in spite of their best efforts, the inability to have an orgasm. It may be difficult for women without clitoral function to reach an orgasm or adequate lubrication, which will reduce the satisfaction they get from their intercourse. Keeping your blood pressure under control enhances your sex life. Treating hypertension, which may be the underlying reason, could result in a more fulfilling and enjoyable sexual experience.

Kidney Failure: Normal Urine is a Bliss

The final organs we will talk about in this part are two that are so essential to life that it is a miracle we were given two! We typically refer to them in the singular tense even though they are two distinct organs. The kidney's main function is to remove excess fluid and toxins from the body by filtering bloodstream toxins and converting serum into urine.

Nonetheless, the kidneys have a network of microscopic branching blood arteries that get smaller as they get deeper into the organs, just like in the brain. Because of their limited arterial network, they are susceptible to harm during a hypertensive emergency. Even while we don't refer to it as a "kidney attack," loss of kidney function while suffering from extremely high blood pressure is essentially what it is. The kidney tissue is harmed in all circumstances and is unable to perform its normal filtering function; these conditions are referred to medically as "acute tubular necrosis" (ATN), "acute kidney injury" (AKI), or "acute renal failure" (ARF).

Common Symptoms and Signs of Acute Kidney Damage
- Insufficient urination or low urine volume
- Face, ankles, and legs swelling
- Extreme exhaustion or fatigue
- Breathlessness.
- Nausea
- Frothy or foamy pee.
- Coma or seizures
- Pain in the chest.

If any of these quickly emerging symptoms appear, you should get emergency medical attention. However, most of the time kidney damage happens with no symptoms experienced by the patient.

When patients are told they have "kidney failure" but are still able to urinate normally, it can be quite confusing for them. The kidneys stop removing toxins from the blood, which is why this occurs. Urine is still produced by them, but they are unable to adequately filter metabolic waste.
As a result, all of the metabolic pollutants are still present and the urine is of poor quality. Fatigue, fogging of the brain, sleeplessness, loss of appetite, and itching might result from this.

Additionally, damaged kidneys can leak proteins into the urine and function as a sieve for certain chemicals. This leads to the passage of minute amounts of protein, which can later be seen in higher proportions on an office urine test.
Eventually, protein can be noted by the naked eye as foam or froth in the urine specimen. Chronic kidney disease has five stages, and the final stage requires intensive treatments— dialysis, kidney transplant, or, in some cases, hospice care.

Chapter 9: Factors affecting Blood Pressure

It is imperative to comprehend the risk factors associated with high blood pressure in order to effectively avoid and treat hypertension. An individual's risk of high blood pressure is influenced by a number of factors. People can decrease their risk and maintain optimal cardiovascular health by making informed decisions based on full awareness of these risk factors.

Age
As we become older, our chance of having high blood pressure rises. Blood arteries may become less elastic over time, which may lead to higher blood pressure and more resistance. Nearly two-thirds of persons over 60 have high blood pressure, according to the American Heart Association, so it's critical to monitor blood pressure levels and establish healthy lifestyle choices early in life.

Gender
Men and women have different prevalence rates of high blood pressure. In general, men are more likely than women to acquire hypertension at a younger age, with the risk

rising sharply after menopause. Premenopausal women are thought to benefit from estrogen's protective effects against hypertension, while these benefits are thought to wane with age. It is imperative to manage blood pressure proactively and implement lifestyle modifications that support heart health, regardless of a person's gender.

Genetics

Genetics and family history can have a big impact on a person's chance of getting high blood pressure. You have an increased chance of getting hypertension if either or both of your parents have the illness. Knowing your family history can help you make more educated decisions regarding your lifestyle and healthcare, even while you cannot change your genetic predisposition.

Lifestyle factors

High blood pressure can result from a variety of lifestyle choices, such as:
- ➢ **Nutrition-less Diet:** Eating a diet heavy in processed foods, and salt, and trans fats can raise blood pressure. A heart-healthy diet can help maintain good cardiovascular health and lower blood pressure. One such diet is the DASH (Dietary Approaches to Stop

Hypertension) diet, which places an emphasis on whole grains, fruits, vegetables, lean proteins, and low-fat dairy products.

➢ **Sedentary Lifestyle:** Sedentary behavior has been linked to elevated blood pressure, weight gain, and a decline in cardiovascular fitness. The heart muscle may weaken as a result of inactivity, which may result in a less effective pumping action and higher blood pressure. Regular physical exercise, such as swimming, cycling, or walking, can help lower blood pressure, strengthen the heart, and enhance general health.

➢ **Excessive alcohol intake:** Drinking too much alcohol can cause weight gain, harm to the liver, and elevated blood pressure. Reducing alcohol consumption can improve general health and help avoid hypertension.

➢ **Stress:** Long-term stress can raise blood pressure by releasing stress hormones, which can narrow blood vessels and increases heartrate. Practicing stress-reduction methods like yoga, meditation, and deep breathing exercises, as well as taking up enjoyable and relaxing hobbies or pastimes, can help control blood pressure and enhance general wellbeing.

Obesity

Being overweight raises the risk of high blood pressure, especially in the belly area. Increased pressure on the artery walls might result from obesity because it makes the heart work harder to pump blood. Furthermore, obesity is frequently linked to other conditions including diabetes, sleep apnea, and high cholesterol, all of which can exacerbate hypertension. Putting a balanced diet and regular exercise into practice while following a weight loss plan can help lower blood pressure and lessen the chance of problems.

Tobacco Consumption

Over time, tobacco use—including smoking and using smokeless tobacco products—can harm the cardiovascular system and temporarily raise blood pressure. Tobacco products contain substances that can constrict blood vessels and stiffen artery walls, raising blood pressure. Reducing tobacco usage and passive smoke exposure can help lower the incidence of hypertension and its related consequences.

Smoking

Smoking can raise blood pressure in the short and long term, much like tobacco usage does. Cigarette nicotine has the ability to momentarily raise blood pressure, quicken heartbeat, and narrow blood vessels. Smoking can cause blood vessel damage and atherosclerosis over time, which raises the risk of hypertension even further. One of the best strategies to reduce blood pressure and enhance cardiovascular health is to give up smoking.

Sleep Apnea

The medical disease known as sleep apnea is characterized by recurrent breathing cessations during sleep, which lower blood oxygen levels. Stress hormones may be released as a result, and blood pressure, heart rate, and heart rate may all rise. Continuous positive airway pressure (CPAP) therapy or other suitable therapies for the treatment of sleep apnea can help lower blood pressure and lessen the risk of problems connected to hypertension.

Kidney Problems

By filtering blood and eliminating excess salt and water, the kidneys are essential in controlling blood pressure. Blood volume and blood pressure can rise when the kidneys are injured or not working properly because they

may not be able to efficiently eliminate extra salt and water from the body.
Blood pressure can be regulated and more kidney damage can be avoided with appropriate renal disease treatment, which includes medication and lifestyle modifications.

Diabetes

Because high blood sugar affects blood arteries and the kidneys, people with diabetes are more likely to develop high blood pressure. Blood arteries that are damaged over time by high blood sugar are more likely to shrink and become less flexible, which raises blood pressure. Diabetes can also affect renal function, which exacerbates hypertension. It is crucial to control diabetes with medicine, food, and exercise in order to keep blood pressure levels within normal range and avoid complications.

By being aware of and taking action against these risk factors, a person's chance of high blood pressure and its related problems can be greatly decreased.

Medication

As a direct side effect or through interactions with other drugs or substances, several medications can raise blood pressure. Decongestants, nonsteroidal anti-inflammatory medicines (NSAIDs), oral contraceptives, and some antidepressants are common medications that might alter blood pressure. Before beginning any new drug, it is important to discuss potential side effects and interactions with your healthcare practitioner. You should also keep a close eye on your blood pressure while taking any medications that may affect it. Discuss potential substitutes or changes to your treatment regimen with your healthcare provider if you believe a medication may be causing your high blood pressure.

We will cover this in detail in the upcoming chapter.

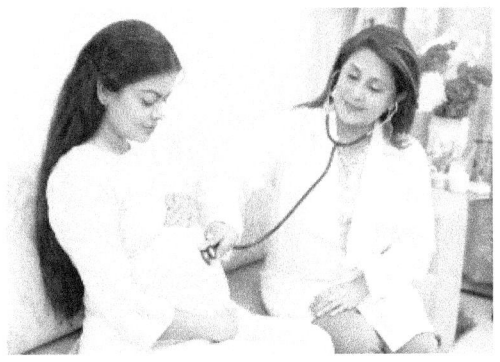

Pregnancy

High blood pressure can develop during pregnancy, either as a pre-existing condition (chronic hypertension) or as a pregnancy-related complication. Pregnant women with high blood pressure are at an increased risk of complications for both themselves and their babies, including preterm birth, low birth weight, and placental abruption. It is essential for women with high blood pressure to receive appropriate prenatal care and work closely with their healthcare providers to monitor and manage their blood pressure throughout pregnancy. In some cases, medication may be prescribed to help control blood pressure levels, while in others, lifestyle changes, such as dietary modifications and exercise may be recommended.

Environmental Factors

Elevated blood pressure has been associated with exposure to specific environmental variables, including noise and air pollution. Prolonged exposure to air pollution, especially particulate matter, can result in oxidative stress and inflammation, which can damage blood vessels and raise blood pressure. In a similar vein, prolonged exposure to loud noises, particularly at night, can raise stress levels and interfere with sleep, both of which can affect blood pressure. Take into consideration employing air purifiers, noise-canceling headphones, or other methods to lessen exposure to air and noise pollution in order to decrease the effects of these environmental factors on blood pressure. Recall that effective hypertension management requires a thorough understanding of blood pressure, its risk factors, and the impact of environmental factors.

People can greatly lower their risk of having high blood pressure and its related consequences by leading a healthy lifestyle, addressing identified risk factors, and being aware of how stress, medicine, and pregnancy affect blood pressure levels.

It is crucial to comprehend how these variables affect blood pressure levels in order to effectively manage and avoid hypertension. Additionally, staying informed and working closely with your healthcare provider will help you determine the best course of action to manage your high blood pressure and enhance your overall health.

Chapter 10: Medications & Prescriptions That Can Cause High Blood Pressure

Certain prescription and over-the-counter drugs can cause blood pressure to rise when used repeatedly. Since it takes time to occur, it is easy to ignore this as a contributing element. If any of the following drugs are on your list, discuss alternative possibilities with your doctor that do not have side effects. Even if stopping these drugs might not always be feasible, you should at least have the conversation and focus more on the lifestyle changes to get rid of the medication.

Sinus and Cold Treatments
- Decongestants work wonders for reducing swollen tissues and relieving nasal or bronchial tube symptoms, but it can also cause blood vessels to shrink, contributing to irregular or fast heartbeats and thereby also increasing blood pressure readings.

Blood Pressure Medications
- Diuretics

  There can be serious electrolyte abnormalities caused by diuretics. Not only may it reduce potassium, but it could also deplete magnesium. Blood pressure can rise due to low magnesium induced by diuretics; however, this side effect can be reversed by taking a magnesium supplement. Adding magnesium also lessens the problem of a potassium shortfall since, in the event that you are obtaining adequate dietary potassium from fruits and vegetables (or a supplement), it will not be absorbed at the cellular level if there is a magnesium deficiency.

> Beta-blockers

Beta-blockers decrease a vital enzyme called Co-Enzyme Q10, which is utilized to address disorders pertaining to the brain, heart, circulatory system, and nerve system. Your body naturally creates this potent antioxidant, sometimes known as the "anti-cellular-rusting" molecule, but as you age, your body produces less of it. Cells require CoQ10 for maintenance and growth, but since certain medications might deplete this enzyme, it's definitely a good idea to check your level of CoQ10 and/or take a supplement if you take a particular prescription.

Melatonin is another hormone that is deficient in beta-blockers. Your brain contains a gland that produces this hormone, which controls sleep and the immune system. It has been demonstrated that beta-blockers lower melatonin synthesis. Your blood pressure will rise in the event that you do not obtain restorative, deep sleep.

Hormones

High blood pressure is also a result of postmenopausal oral hormone replacement therapy or birth control tablets. Hormone suppositories and lotions are less risky and safer alternatives.

Oral Estrogen

High blood pressure has been linked to oral estrogen.
It takes a lot of B vitamins to digest and get rid of all kinds of estrogen. This implies that if you use hormone replacement treatment or take birth control pills, you run the risk of developing a B vitamin deficit. For those who take hormones, make sure you are taking enough vitamin Bs because low levels of these vitamins might cause blood pressure and stickiness.

Testosterone boosters

Testosterone boosters may cause hypertension. Younger men are more susceptible to this effect than older men are, as are athletes who abuse testosterone to boost their performance. During their gender-affirming therapy, transgender women might see a decrease in blood pressure, while transgender men might experience an increase. The symptoms of low testosterone can affect both men and women. Hopefully, if you experience low testosterone symptoms, your doctor is checking for this. A high dosage of testosterone can elevate blood pressure and should be lowered, thus it's important to pay close attention to dosage and adverse effects. All patients who need hormone therapy should generally undergo regular blood pressure checks.

Anti-Inflammatory Pain Medications

Non-steroidal anti-inflammatory drug (NSAID) is a class of pharmaceuticals that is well known for destroying kidney cells and accelerating chronic renal disease in addition to increasing blood pressure. This category includes both prescription and over-the-counter options, so let your doctors know if you take prescription arthritis or pain relievers or if you self-medicate with aspirin.

In general, homeopathic and herbal pain relievers don't seem to have an impact on blood pressure.

Steroids

We occasionally administer steroid dosage packs or cortisone shots for joint discomfort, sinus infections, or skin rashes, while they are most frequently used for life-threatening illnesses like allergic reactions and asthma attacks. Although steroids can significantly lessen discomfort, among its many possible side effects include fluid retention, electrolyte imbalances, mood swings, high blood sugar, and elevated blood pressure. Additional blood pressure monitoring is advised if you must take them.

Antidepressants

High blood pressure can be brought on by or made worse by almost all drug classes used to treat long-term anxiety, depression, or OCD (obsessive-compulsive disorder). Although, there are class of medications which are exception to this rule. So, please consult your physician in this regard.

Antipsychotic Medications

Bipolar disorder or treatment-resistant depression are the illnesses for which these medications are used more frequently. Fortunately, you can lower your need for these drugs by adhering to the foundational principles of wellbeing. Lower doses have less of an impact on blood pressure and fewer negative effects than higher levels.

Immunosuppressive Treatment

You will probably be taking an immunosuppressant medication to avoid transplant rejection if you have received an organ transplant and have been granted a second chance at life. These medications are also prescribed in the event of certain autoimmune diseases. Since discontinuing these medications is usually not an option, it is necessary to be mindful of the impact on blood pressure, to monitor closely, and occasionally to start BP medication.

Biologic Medications

These are the drugs that are the subject of all TV advertisements. They represent a significant advancement in the treatment of inflammatory diseases like psoriasis and rheumatoid arthritis, as well as those with genetically predisposed forms of high cholesterol. Home blood pressure monitoring should probably be part of your plan as hypertension is a side effect for some of you who need these medications.

Cholesterol-Lowering Medications

These drugs have been proven to deplete specific minerals, just like beta-blockers. As the statins are metabolized, CoQ10, vitamin D, vitamin K, and selenium are all decreased; any of these deficits can impact blood pressure and cardiovascular risk. To achieve the benefits of the drug without the hazards, levels must be watched carefully, and supplements must frequently be taken.

Herbal Supplements

Not to be overlooked, some herbal supplements purchased over-the-counter can also increase blood pressure! We must honor and respect the plants and herbs we use for their medical worth and be aware of any potential adverse effects related to blood pressure, even though they are typically safer and more tolerated than pharmaceutical drugs. Certain stimulants that are frequently included in formulas for energy drinks or diet plans may raise blood pressure.

There are substitutes for these herbs. Bach Flower treatments soothe anxiety and fear. Herbal forms have more adverse effects on the cardiovascular system than do homeopathic ones. Certain drugs have the potential to create nutrient deficits in addition to hypertension.

Chapter 11: Benefits, Risks and Side-effects of BP Medications

Benefits
- If untreated, high blood pressure can result in a number of serious health problems, including heart attacks, strokes, renal disease, and vision loss. By correctly treating the disease, blood pressure medications help reduce the likelihood of these problems.
- People who have their blood pressure under control can live longer, healthier lives without always worrying about the possible issues that could arise from high blood pressure. By lessening the strain on the heart and blood vessels, blood pressure medications not only lower blood pressure but also improve heart health in general.

Risks
- Blood pressure medications might have negative effects, just like any other medication. These could be modest and transient or more severe and long-lasting.
- Hypotension, or abnormally low blood pressure, can occasionally result from

blood pressure medications lowering blood pressure too much. Shock, fainting, or dizziness could come from this.
➢ When blood pressure medications are taken with other prescription drugs, dietary supplements, or herbal therapies, there can occasionally be negative interactions that decrease the effectiveness of the treatment or result in negative side effects.

Side-effects

The typical adverse effects of blood pressure medications differ based on the drug in question and the patient's reaction to the treatment. Typical adverse effects include the following:

➢ **Dizziness:** This can happen when blood pressure falls too quickly, which results in a brief decrease in blood supply to the brain.
➢ **Headaches:** When starting a new drug or changing the dosage, some people may have headaches as a side effect of blood pressure medications.
➢ **Fatigue:** Feelings of fatigue or exhaustion may be brought on by certain

blood pressure drugs, especially beta-blockers.
- **Gastrointestinal problems:** Some blood pressure drugs might cause nausea, diarrhea, or constipation as adverse effects.
- **Dry cough:** It has been shown that ACE inhibitors (angiotensin-converting enzyme used to treat and manage cardiovascular conditions) can give some people a chronic dry cough. An ARB (angiotensin receptor blockers) could be suitable substitute for these patients. Please consult your healthcare professional in this regard.
- **Insomnia:** Some blood pressure drugs, such beta-blockers, might make it harder to get asleep or stay asleep.
- **Lower extremity swelling:** Calcium channel blockers may result in fluid retention, which can exacerbate swelling in the legs, ankles, or foot.
- **Erectile dysfunction:** Men's erectile dysfunction may be exacerbated by certain blood pressure medications, including beta-blockers and diuretics.
- **Weight gain:** Some blood pressure medications, particularly beta-blockers, may cause weight gain due to fluid retention or changes in metabolism.

- **Skin rash:** People on blood pressure medications can have skin rashes or photosensitivity.

Talking to your healthcare practitioner about any adverse effects you have is crucial. A medication's side effects can frequently be controlled or eliminated by changing the dosage or prescription.

Chapter 12: When Do You Actually Need Medicine for High Blood Pressure?

Numerous criteria, such as your blood pressure readings, general health, and the existence of additional risk factors or illnesses, play a role in determining whether you require medication for high blood pressure.

Your BP is consistently 140/90 or higher

Healthcare professionals utilize predetermined criteria to assess if a patient needs medication for hypertension. Generally, your doctor may think about writing a prescription for medication if your blood pressure regularly registers at 140/90 mm Hg or above.

Lifestyle changes are not helping you in controlling elevated BP

Your doctor could advise lifestyle modifications, such as adopting a healthier diet, getting regular exercise, losing weight, managing your stress, and cutting back on alcohol and tobacco use, if your blood pressure is only slightly raised. It could be required to take medication if these lifestyle changes are not enough to decrease blood pressure.

Remember that it takes time to make changes to your lifestyle and if you can control your blood pressure through this step, it is undoubtedly the best step you are taking for longevity and healthier life.

You already have other medical conditions

Even if your blood pressure is only slightly elevated, your healthcare practitioner may prescribe medicine to aggressively manage it if you have other health concerns including diabetes, renal disease, or heart disease. The goal of this strategy is to lower the chance of problems brought on by high blood pressure.

You're an older individual

Given the increased risk of issues with aging, older adults may need to take medication to control their blood pressure.

You have a family history

In the event that high blood pressure or associated issues run in your family, your doctor might suggest medication as a prophylactic step.

If you fall into one or more criteria mentioned above, it's best and important to collaborate closely with your healthcare professional. The more information you will be able to provide to your healthcare professional clearly, the better advice and treatment can be expected in return.

Chapter 13: Combination Therapy for Managing High BP

Often, controlling high blood pressure necessitates a multifaceted approach that includes both medicine and lifestyle changes. By taking care of your food, exercise routine, stress levels, and smoking habits, you can lower your blood pressure and reduce the likelihood of problems from this illness.

Nevertheless, there are situations in which changing your lifestyle on its own might not be enough to lower your blood pressure to a safe level. In certain situations, taking medication to help reduce your blood pressure can be recommended. For you, your healthcare professional is the primary source of advice regarding which medicine or combination of medications is best. Your medical history, risk factors, and general state of health will all be considered.

Using a combination of two or more medications can help manage blood pressure and increase medication tolerance for treating high blood pressure. Raising the dosage of one drug alone may not be as successful in decreasing blood pressure as using two drugs with distinct mechanisms of action.

Additionally, this strategy makes it possible to utilize smaller dosages of each medication, which may minimize side effects and encourage adherence to the recommended course of care.

Studies have shown that combination therapy can assist people with high blood pressure better control their disease, often outperforming single-drug therapy. Combination therapy for high blood pressure can produce impressive outcomes, but finding the right medication combination for you requires careful collaboration with your healthcare professional. It is crucial to remember that not all medications can be mixed together safely. In fact, some combinations can have negative impacts on your health, such as interactions or side effects.

Let's examine a few of the factors that make combo therapy a more sensible strategy in order to comprehend its advantages:

Improved Regulation of Blood Pressure

Combination therapy can offer a more thorough method of treating high blood pressure by focusing on several components of the blood pressure regulation system. For instance, combining a beta-blocker, which lowers heart rate and contraction force, with a diuretic, which eliminates extra fluid from the body, can lead to more effective blood pressure control than using either medication alone.

Reduced Side Effects

Combination therapy helps minimize adverse effects because it frequently calls for lowering the dosages of individual medications. Additionally, patients can handle the medications more easily at lower doses, which increases the chance that they will follow the treatment plan.

Combination Medications

For some people, taking many drugs might be difficult, but combination therapy can make it easier. Fixed-dose combination tablets, which combine two or more blood pressure-lowering drugs into one tablet, are sold by numerous pharmaceutical companies. Patients may find it easier to take their prescriptions as directed as a result, which may enhance treatment compliance and blood pressure regulation in general.

Faster Reduction in Blood Pressure

Combination therapy may sometimes cause blood pressure to drop more quickly. For people with extremely high blood pressure or those who are at a higher risk of developing consequences from high blood pressure, this can be especially helpful.

Challenges Associated with Combination Therapy

It's important to understand that combination therapy may have certain disadvantages despite its advantages. Among the difficulties this strategy presents are:

Interactions Between Drugs
When several medications are used together, there is a higher chance of drug interactions, which can have negative side effects or lower the effectiveness of the medications. To reduce this risk, it is essential to discuss with your healthcare practitioner all of the prescriptions you use, including over-the-counter medications and vitamins.

A Higher Price
The cost of treatment may be a deterrent for some people if they take many medications. Long-term savings on complications and better blood pressure management could, however, more than make up for these expenses.

The Intricacy of the Therapy

Taking several drugs at once can be challenging, especially for elderly or cognitively impaired people. Working collaboratively with your healthcare practitioner, you should devise techniques to streamline your treatment plan and guarantee appropriate drug administration and adherence.

Strategies to Overcome the Challenges of Combination Therapy

In order to surmount these obstacles and optimize the advantages of combination therapy, contemplate the subsequent tactics:

Consult your Healthcare Practitioner Regularly

Keep lines of communication open with your healthcare practitioner regarding your symptoms, worries, and prescription drugs. This will make it easier for them to comprehend your particular requirements and track your development, modifying your treatment plan as necessary.

Following Your Treatment Regimen

It is essential to adhere to your doctor's advised treatment plan in order to achieve ideal blood pressure control. Recall to take your drugs exactly as prescribed, and let your doctor know if you have any adverse affects or have trouble adhering to your regimen.

Frequent Blood Pressure Checks

You and your doctor can evaluate the efficacy of your treatment plan and make any required modifications if you routinely monitor your blood pressure, either at home or at visits. Monitoring your blood pressure at home can be quite useful for determining how changes in medicine and lifestyle affect your blood pressure.

Lifestyle Changes

Continue to place a high priority on lifestyle modifications such as stress reduction, regular exercise, a good diet, and quitting smoking in addition to combination therapy. These changes can enhance your general health and well-being in addition to lowering your blood pressure.

Remain Knowledgeable and Proactive

Learn about high blood pressure and the

several drugs that are used to treat it. Making proactive and educated decisions regarding your health can facilitate meaningful conversations with your healthcare practitioner.

To sum up, combination therapy can be a very successful strategy for controlling high blood pressure, especially when combined with lifestyle changes. You can take charge of your high blood pressure and strive toward a healthier future by collaborating closely with your healthcare practitioner, keeping a close eye on your blood pressure, and following your treatment plan. Keep in mind that every person's experience with high blood pressure is different, and it may take some time to find the right mix of prescription drugs and lifestyle modifications. Nevertheless, with perseverance and the help of your medical team, you can improve your blood pressure control and your general quality of life.

Chapter 14: Avoid Interference with Other Medicines

It's critical to be proactive and keep lines of communication open with your healthcare team in order to prevent interactions between high blood pressure drugs and other substances. The following useful advice will help reduce possible interactions and guarantee that your high blood pressure is safely and effectively managed:

Keep Your Healthcare Updated

Make sure all of your medical professionals are aware of everything you take, including vitamins, nutritional and herbal supplements, prescription and over-the-counter medications, and prescription pharmaceuticals. They will be better able to assess any possible interactions and suggest appropriate courses of action as a result.

Consult Before Taking New Medicine

Ask important questions, such if the new drug will interact with your current drugs, when is the ideal time to take it, and whether there are any probable adverse effects, to your pharmacist or healthcare provider before starting any new prescription.

Label Reading

Go over the labels of all the prescription and over-the-counter medications you take with great care. Important information regarding possible interactions and negative effects is frequently included on labels.

Single Pharmacy for Records

If you fill all of your prescriptions at the same pharmacy, the pharmacist will have a comprehensive record of all of your drugs, which will make it simpler for them to spot possible interactions and offer individualized advice.

Recall that controlling high blood pressure is a continuous process, so it's critical to continue being proactive, knowledgeable, and involved in your treatment regimen. You may improve blood pressure control and have a healthier future by using these helpful suggestions and the assistance of your healthcare team.

Chapter 15: Follow-Up Questions to Ask Your Healthcare Professional

It's critical to have an honest discussion with your healthcare practitioner before beginning any high blood pressure medication to make sure the drug of choice is appropriate for your needs and safe. Here are some crucial questions you should think about asking your physician or pharmacist to help direct your conversation:

- ➢ **What is the main purpose of this medicine?**
  Inquire with your healthcare practitioner about the drug's intended use, mechanism of action, and anticipated advantages for controlling your blood pressure.

- ➢ **Should I alter my lifestyle in any way while taking this medication?**
  Talk about any suggested changes to your diet, exercise regimen, or other aspects of your lifestyle that could support your treatment plan for high blood pressure.

- ➢ **When and how should I take this medication?**
  Find out the right amount to take, when

to take it, and if you should take the medication with or without meals. For optimal absorption and efficacy, this information is essential.

- ➢ **Are there potential adverse reactions or incompatibilities with food or dietary supplements?**
  Recognize any interactions between particular foods, drinks, or dietary supplements and probable adverse effects that may impact the safety or efficacy of the medicine.

- ➢ **Does this medication interfere with other medications if you are consuming other medicines?**
  Talk to your doctor about any possible interactions with other medications you are taking, and find out about any red flags for bad drug interactions.

- ➢ **How much time will it take for the drug to start working?**
  Find out from your doctor how long it should take for the medicine to start affecting your blood pressure.

- ➢ **How often should I check my blood pressure and how can I tell if the medicine is working?**
  Find out how to assess the efficacy of

your prescription and the ideal interval for taking your blood pressure.

> **What safety measures ought I to follow when taking this medication?**
Recognize any special safety measures that apply to you while taking the drug, such as avoiding certain meals, beverages, or activities.

> **How should I proceed if I inadvertently take more dosage or forget to take a dose?**
Find out what to do if you inadvertently take more medication than is recommended or forget to take a dose.

> **When is the best time for me to get a follow-up appointment to check my blood pressure and see how well the medicine is working?**
Choose the best time for a follow-up visit with your healthcare practitioner to assess your blood pressure and talk about the efficacy of the drug.

You can better control your high blood pressure and lower your risk of consequences by asking these important questions and remaining knowledgeable about your medication and any potential interactions. Recall that obtaining ideal blood pressure control and enhancing your general health depend on your active participation in your treatment plan and your open communication with your healthcare team.

Chapter 16: What if Your Left and Right Sides Have Different BP Readings

Did you know? - You can have different blood pressure readings between your right and your left sides? And not by a little bit, either, but as much as 15 mmHg, or more.

Difference of ~5mmHg
Your high blood pressure is actually a cardiovascular issue if it is elevated on both sides and the difference is only roughly 5 mmHg.

Difference of ~15mmHg
If there is a significant discrepancy (remember, significant means at least 15 mmHg) between your left and right sides, your issue is neurological rather than cardiovascular. The brain stem contains the portion of the brain that regulates blood pressure on both sides.

Testing the other side is crucial if one side has elevated blood pressure. In the event when the blood pressure on your other side is normal, neurological treatment is what you should receive. not directed at the heart. A sizable proportion of people are misdiagnosed as having high blood pressure and receiving incorrect treatment when, in reality, their issue is with the brain stem.

Chapter 17: Workouts for High Blood Pressure

Your doctor will simply say, "You should exercise. It is beneficial to you."
But most of the times no further information is provided beyond that.

Important details are needed like:
- Should you do strength training, cardio, or stretching?
- What number of days in a week?
- What should be the level of intensity or maximum heart rate during workout?
- For what length of time?

FITT Principle
So, remember the **FITT** principle to plan your exercise regimen.
- Frequency
- Intensity
- Time
- Type

Frequency
- If your lifestyle has been sedentary till now, start with 3-5 days per week.

Intensity

If you have not been exercising, you should not increase your intensity from level 0 to level 5. An elderly person who leads a sedentary lifestyle has a relatively weaker heart than someone who exercises often and leads an active lifestyle.

Hence, if you follow a regular routine, begin at a low intensity, give your body and heart time to adjust, and then progressively increase it over the course of the following few months as you go from low to moderate and finally high.

- Start with completing 5000 steps per day if you don't even do that currently.
- Follow this for a week and then increase it to 7000-8000 steps for a week.
- Further increase it to 10000 steps for the next week.
- If you are comfortably able to do this now, add brisk walks, replace escalators with stairs, or jog at a low pace.
- Now, you are slightly active and you should add light bodyweight exercises like squats, plank hold, or use resistance bands to strengthen your muscles.

- Gradually you can increase the intensity and add cycling, running, weight training.
- Once you are comfortable with moderate intensity for 12 weeks or so, without impacting your energy levels and blood pressure readings, you can further increase the intensity and add some sport, HIIT (High Intensity Interval Training).

So, you don't have to lift very heavy weights or push yourself to an extent that you invite injuries and have to take rest for more time. As we age, we are more prone to injuries than young people!

Instead, you can add more volume to increase intensity like adding more reps or sets or decreasing rest time between sets. This will still increase your muscle size (hypertrophy) provided your nutrition is balanced.

The maximum heart rate during workout for an individual having hypertension can be determined below equation:

$162 - (0.7 \times age)$ = estimated maximum heart rate (HRmax)

Time

If you are a beginner, start with 20-30 minutes. Even 20 minutes might be too difficult for you if your current lifestyle has been inactive. Don't worry, just get up and move!

You will definitely see some progress within a week or so if you are taking steps toward lifestyle changes.

Gradually, increase the time to 30 minutes if 20-25 minutes doesn't challenge you over the time. Similarly, if 30 minutes are not challenging enough, you can increase it to 45 minutes or 60 minutes eventually.

60 minutes is very decent and enough if your intensity level is moderate and you are regular like 4-5 days a week.

You can definitely increase beyond 60 minutes as well, but I would suggest you to check other factors first like

How much rest time are you taking between the sets? Is there a scope to reduce your rest period? (Like bring it down to 30 seconds or when you can catch back your breath)

Are the weights you are using challenging enough for the sets?

Do you sweat during workout?

Do you feel that your heart is elevated?

Because if you are comfortably exercising for 60 minutes daily, your workout is not challenging enough, and if it is challenging, and still you have the capacity to increase the overall time period over 60 minutes, then you are not a beginner anymore.

Type

Individual with hypertension should engage themselves in:
- **Cardiovascular activities**
  150 minutes of moderate-intense exercise
  OR
  75 minutes of strenuous activity
  OR
  any combination of the two.
- **Resistance Training**
  Exercise at a moderate to high intensity twice a week.
  Gradually boost the intensity, warm up, and cool down.

Concurrent training, sometimes referred to as circuit training, is another option available. This approach might be the most effective in lowering blood pressure and lowering the risk of hypertension. Its overall effect on the risk factors for cardiovascular disease is better.

Before starting a weight-lifting program, individuals with blood pressure more than 160/100 mm Hg should speak with their doctor because high resistance can momentarily raise blood pressure. Instead of performing strenuous overhead lifts, people should alternate between upper and lower body workouts.

It is better to start your fitness journey in the guidance of a personal trainer at least in the initial few weeks or months.
A personal trainer will not only help you in pushing your limits but will also keep a check on your posture or form during workouts which is very crucial to stay away from injuries.
You will also get to know the exercises related to each muscle group or body part and how should you plan your workouts.

Instead of surrendering yourself to a personal trainer, I would suggest you to stay active, learn and understand what workouts they are providing you on which days, how many sets or reps are they advising and ask them questions so that in the long run, you can become independent in designing and planning your own workouts and save money on trainers.

A beginner or an intermediate person can also refer my book 'Add Fitness to Lifestyle' that would certainly help you give a direction and

clear a lot of questions regarding workout and lifestyle.
https://www.amazon.com/Add-Fitness-Lifestyle-Training-Passively-ebook/dp/B0CHR4WXJC/

Other Factors During Workout

Controlled Breathing

Do not hold your breath during workout! Holding the breath during workouts raises intravenous pressure on veins and runs the risk of damage and syncope.
Furthermore, it is recommended that people with high BP refrain from performing the Valsalva technique. Some weight lifters employ this technique to maximize force generation by engaging the core.

Valsalva maneuver
When your heart is racing too quickly, you can slow it down by using the Valsalva breathing technique. It is carried out by making a strong endeavor to exhale against a closed airway, which is typically accomplished by pinching one's nose together, closing one's lips, and forcing air out as if inflating a balloon. It is possible to utilize variations of this maneuver to clear the sinuses and ears or to examine cardiac function and autonomic nervous system regulation during a medical checkup.

Warm-Up

For patients with high blood pressure, warming up is crucial because it permits the blood arteries to gradually widen to accept increased blood flow. People should be able to reach their desired heart rate with the aid of a slow warm-up. It is essential to give at least ten minutes, if not more if they haven't been active recently.

Cooldown

Just as crucial is the cooldown that follows the workout. It's crucial to resist letting the client end engagement right away. We need to gradually return our heart rate to pre-exercise levels by incorporating yoga or flexibility exercises. In addition, a suitable cooldown will reduce muscle soreness post workout.

Exercise is an Overall Game Changer

Heart is a muscle, and muscles grow stronger with exercise. Engaging in regular physical activity helps our heart circulate blood throughout the body more efficiently, which lessens the load on this important organ.

Frequent exercise improves heart's ability to pump blood, which lowers the pressure on the arteries. Over time, this heart-strengthening

impact may result in a long-lasting drop in blood pressure and resting heart rate.
By increasing levels of good cholesterol (HDL) and lowering levels of bad cholesterol (LDL), exercise also helps to improve lipid profiles. This equilibrium can lower the risk of atherosclerosis and heart disease by preventing the accumulation of cholesterol in the arteries.

Moreover, the enhanced circulation promotes the healing and growth of the cells, further improving the function and structure of the cardiovascular system.

Regular physical activity improves the body's sensitivity to insulin, reducing the risk of type 2 diabetes—a significant risk factor for heart disease. For those already living with diabetes, exercise helps manage the condition, lessening its impact on heart health.

In short, exercise helps in decreasing your blood pressure and helps you to stay away from other medical conditions and leads to longevity.

Chapter 18: Nutrition for High Blood Pressure

Although, there are many diets and terms that you might hear but more or less they have a common goal and that is change in lifestyle by:
- Limiting to restricting processed food
- Limiting sugar and red meat
- Adding fruits and vegetables in your diet (eat more fiber)
- Increasing lean protein in your diet

One of the most recommended diets in such cases is DASH (Dietary Approaches to Stop Hypertension) diet.

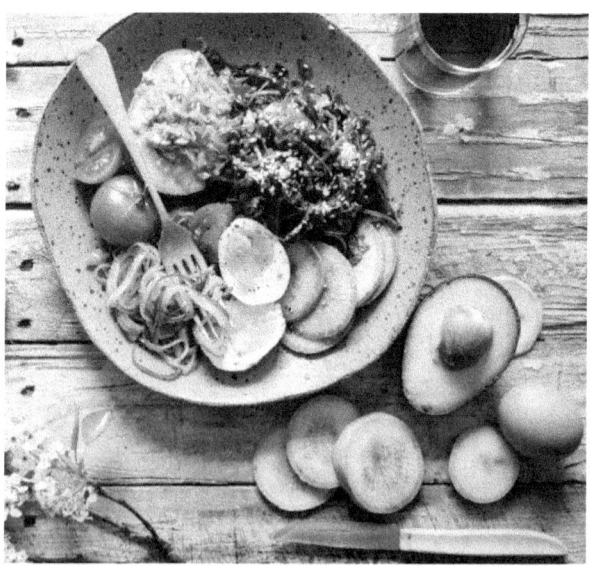

DASH Diet

Anyone with high blood pressure is the main target audience for the DASH diet, which aims to lower hypertension with the least amount of medication or none at all.

The diet is easy to follow. There are no specific dietary limits; instead, there is a weekly plan consisting of X healthy calories per day, where X is your nutritionist's recommended calorie intake.

The diet eschews fatty meats, full-fat dairy, coconut and palm oil, and sweets in favor of low-fat dairy, fish, poultry, legumes, nuts, and vegetable oils. A normal sodium intake of up to 2,300 milligrams per day or a reduced sodium intake of up to 1,500 milligrams per day can both be followed when following the DASH diet.

The DASH diet recommends that 55 percent of daily Calories come from carbohydrates, approximately 27 percent from unsaturated fats, 6 percent from saturated fats, and 18 percent from protein.

Tips include filling the plate with colorful, whole foods and including two or more servings of fruits and vegetables per meal, with a particular emphasis on dark, leafy green vegetables. In addition to lowering blood pressure, the DASH diet has other health benefits: prevention of bone loss, improved cardiovascular health, and weight loss or maintenance.

Food Items	Servings/Day
Fresh Fruits & Vegetables	4 to 5
Grains	6 to 8
Lean Protein	Upto 6
Nuts, Seeds or Legumes	0.5 to 0.75
Fats and Sweets	Very Limited (avoid if possible)

Mediterranean Diet

People who live in numerous Mediterranean countries, such as Greece, Spain, and Italy, have reduced rates of chronic health conditions, according to study on global health and wellness. This is commonly ascribed to the local way of life.

The World Health Organization (WHO) and the United Nations Educational, Scientific, and Cultural Organization (UNESCO) have included the benefits of the Mediterranean diet to their list of intangible cultural heritages because of how universally acknowledged and accepted the diet is. The listing attempts to safeguard the "food-related skills, harvesting, cooking, and consumption" that the diet encourages.

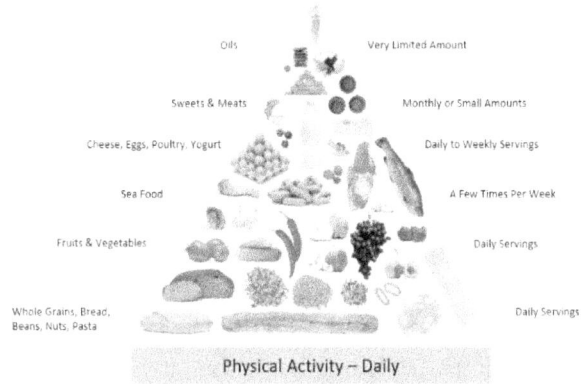

The Mediterranean diet calls for small amounts of red meat and moderate portion of fish, poultry, eggs, dairy, fruits, vegetables, whole grains, legumes, potatoes, nuts, seeds, olive oil.

The Mediterranean population may have lower rates of chronic illness and cardiovascular disease in large part because of their high intake of heart-healthy omega-3 fatty acids. People who are at high risk of heart attack, stroke, or arterial plaques are frequently advised to follow this diet.

This diet is composed of light, fresh foods that are both nourishing and delicious. This eventually causes a natural reduction in caloric consumption, which aids in weight loss. According to studies, a Mediterranean diet can significantly lower the risk of type 2 diabetes and lower the risk of cardiovascular disease by up to 30%.
But, do not forget to include proteins in your daily diet since lack of protein would make you lose more muscle mass than fat mass and you will eventually degrade your metabolism (BMR).

It is difficult for a beginner to completely change their lifestyle suddenly without guidance. The nutrition topic is quite vast and there is a lot to explain about the science behind it and how to make changes in your eating habits gradually to adopt a healthy lifestyle without totally restricting the items you love or following a very restrictive diet where you give up after a few weeks or so.

It is always advisable to kickstart your journey under the professional guidance. I suggest you to consult your Nutritionist in this regard, while if you have a very limited to no idea on how to kickstart, my last book over Amazon 'Eat Mindfully Cheat Wisely' will definitely

provide you immense information and direction on how to kickstart your nutrition journey.
https://www.amazon.com/Eat-Mindfully-Cheat-Wisely-Explaining/dp/B0CM9HTJ5X/

Chapter 19: Factors that might help you in Quick Fixes for Extreme Cases

Your blood pressure may occasionally increase for recognized or unexplained reasons. Medication is one option, although it frequently takes some time for it to work. There are several methods that, in less than five minutes, can drop your blood pressure by as much as 10–40 points!

These can nearly always keep you out of danger if you forget your medication, had a stressful or frightening experience, or consumed anything that raised your blood pressure. However, they are not a replacement for quality medical treatment.

Breathing Techniques

There are numerous variations of breathwork patterns. I advise you to try each one. Select a technique you enjoy and use it often. Some will seem effortless and natural, while others could make you feel constrictive. The effect is more long-lasting the more often you apply them.

- **Breathing in waves: five in, five out**
  Take five deep breaths through your nose, then release the air for six to seven

seconds with your lips slightly pursed. Take five deep breaths, followed by six or seven exhaled. Repeat four or six times, or until you start to feel more at ease and relaxed.

It has been demonstrated that this technique increases heart rate variability and lowers blood pressure.

- ➤ **Box Breathing**

  Here's another method for lowering blood pressure that has been scientifically proved. Take a seat in a quiet area and place one hand on your belly and one on your chest. When you breathe, try to bring your diaphragm down so that your belly hand moves more than your chest hand. You inhale for four seconds, hold your breath for four seconds, exhale for four seconds, then hold your breath for four seconds when using this approach. Inhale, hold, exhale, and hold again. For four to five minutes, repeat about fifteen to twenty times. Navy seals practice box breathing to maintain their composure and awareness.

Empty Your Bladder

A full bladder can elevate your score by ten to fifteen points, and the effect can linger for up to three hours. If you need to urinate, don't make the mistake of taking your blood pressure!

Acupressure

Our second quick remedy for high blood pressure is from the acupuncture tradition. We are aware that communication occurs through our skin and neurological system, and that our bodies function as a switchboard or electrical grid. Some pressure spots on your extremities have been discovered by practitioners as having the ability to instantly reduce blood pressure when stimulated.

> ➢ **The tip of the middle finger of hand**
> On your fingertip is one of these spots. Given how simple it is to locate, it is helpful to be aware of this pressure point. It is located on the tips of the middle fingers on both hands; to locate it, recall "the tip of the middle of the middle." Press this point with an orange stick, chopstick, or retracted ink pen, and hold it for at least a minute to reduce blood pressure and relieve palpitations and the sensation of being hot. Remember that this is a short-term

solution to regain control of your blood pressure when you aren't taking your medicine; it is not a cure for persistently high blood pressure.

➢ **Top of the foot: Along the line between the toe and the second finger**
This point lies on the top of the foot, is excellent for relieving tense energy and treating headaches that originate at the temples. Additionally, it might reduce blood pressure. Draw a line with your finger between the toe and second finger. This point of acupressure is located in the tiny indentation right before your finger touches the bone. Apply deep pressure for approximately three seconds with the same retractable pen, and then take a five-second break. After two minutes of repetition, massage the opposite foot in the same manner.

Meditation
Meditation is another fast blood pressure remedy. You can practice meditation for free and in any location! It takes time to adapt and does not happen all at once. You improve with each training session, and your skills accumulate over time. However, it genuinely helps to lower anxiety and relieve tension. If

you can, try to fit in five minutes each morning and, if not, add a few minutes here and there throughout the week.

Side-Lying

Changing your body's position is another way to quickly reduce your blood pressure. For at least five minutes, lie on your left side (this can be paired with the previously indicated breathwork numbers).

If you are pregnant, sleeping on your left side of the bed is the best position for optimal health and relaxation. The blood veins in our chest and abdomen, somewhat to the right of our spine, are responsible for returning deoxygenated blood to our heart. Sleeping on our right side increases the pressure on those blood vessels. This essentially makes it more difficult for our organs to cleanse and for the heart to pump enough blood to meet the body's needs.

Sleeping on your left side slightly lessens the workload on your heart. Try bending your knees or placing a pillow between your thighs and knees if this causes pain in your back or knees.

Chapter 20: Effects of Caffeine on High Blood Pressure

Although caffeine's effects on blood pressure are well-established and evident in the short term, its long-term effects are less obvious. Studies vary in their conclusions; some point to a possible minor increase in the risk of hypertension with regular coffee use, while others show that the body can eventually become tolerant to these effects. Further investigation is required to completely comprehend the long-term consequences of regular coffee consumption.

It's critical to monitor and control blood pressure in people with hypertension. Although there isn't a universal solution, people with high blood pressure should take their particular situation into account when determining how much coffee to drink. While some people may have little to no influence on their blood pressure, others may be more susceptible to the effects of coffee and should limit their intake. To decide on the best course of action, speaking with a healthcare practitioner is advised.

Decaffeinated coffee is a good substitute for those who want to reduce the amount of caffeine in their coffee because it has a much lower caffeine content than regular coffee. For some people, even decaf coffee can nevertheless result in a tiny, transient rise in blood pressure. It's crucial to pay attention to your body's reaction while deciding if decaf coffee is a good choice.

If you discover that drinking coffee considerably increases your blood pressure or makes your hypertension worse, you should think about cutting back or giving it up. Reduce your coffee intake gradually to avoid experiencing withdrawal symptoms including headaches, exhaustion, and irritability.

Alternatives
Many substitutes for coffee might offer a reassuring ritual without raising blood pressure for people who want to cut back or give it up. Herbal teas with flavors and warmth (such peppermint or chamomile) are free of caffeine.

Green tea has more antioxidants and less caffeine than coffee, even though it still contains some of the same stimulants. Chicory root coffee is a caffeine-free alternative that tastes and smells just like coffee. It might be a good replacement for coffee. Making educated decisions about your coffee intake requires an understanding of the link between blood pressure and caffeine.

Finding the ideal balance for your health and wellbeing requires you to pay attention to your body, speak with a healthcare provider, and consider your options.

Chapter 21: Other Helpful Factors

Sleep

The most crucial element when it comes to the body starting vital maintenance processes is sleep. Hormones are controlled, muscles are rebuilt, and tissues are restored. The brain cleans away poisons, analyzes and consolidates memories, and rejuvenates itself for the next day as we sleep.

It is essential for preserving mental clarity, emotional stability, and physical health.

Our blood pressure and pulse rate drop dramatically when we get good sleep, providing our cardiovascular system with a much-needed respite. The heart and circulatory system can also heal from any harm done by the stresses of the day during this restorative phase. Furthermore, a proper sleep schedule can help lower inflammation and raise cholesterol, two factors that are critical for preserving heart health and lowering the risk of cardiovascular illnesses.

Conversely, inadequate sleep or diseases related to sleep, such as sleep apnea, can negatively impact heart health. An irregular heartbeat, raised stress hormones, elevated blood pressure, and increased inflammation can all result from these problems. These effects can raise the risk of cardiac disorders such as hypertension, stroke, and heart failure in addition to exerting stress on the heart.

Steer clear of caffeinated drinks later in the day. If caffeine is taken after midnight, it may remain elevated in your blood for 6–8 hours, which could interfere with your sleep.

Stress Management

When you're in a stressful scenario, your system releases stress chemicals like cortisol and adrenaline. These hormones drive the heart rate to rise, the energy level to spike, and the blood vessels to constrict—all survival strategies meant to keep us alive in the event of a perceived threat.

Persistently elevated blood pressure might result from these physiological alterations being maintained by chronic stress.

Stress can be reduced by meditation or physical activity such as jogging, cycling, swimming, or any sport.

Quit Smoking

We've already talked about how smoking causes high blood pressure. They may cause damage to blood arteries, lessening their flexibility and increasing the likelihood that fatty deposits will build up inside of them, eventually leading to atherosclerosis, a major risk factor for hypertension.

The chance of a heart attack begins to decrease a few weeks after stopping. The increased risk of coronary heart disease is halved after approximately a year, compared to smokers. The risk of stroke also decreases to that of a nonsmoker over a period of 5 to 15 years.

Limit Alcohol

Blood pressure can be directly impacted by alcohol. It will dilate blood arteries when used intoxicatingly, but when ingested in larger quantities, it will promote the production of hormones that narrow blood vessels. Blood pressure will immediately rise as a result of this.

While this effect wears off quickly for normal drinkers, heavy drinkers may have a persistent rise in blood pressure that eventually results in hypertension.

Certain demographics may experience negative effects from even moderate alcohol intake. For example, alcohol should not be consumed by those who have been diagnosed with specific heart problems, such as heart failure or irregular heart rhythms. Alcohol can aggravate these diseases by interfering with the heart's regular function.

Chapter 21: Closure

The rising hypertension cases are alarming since high blood pressure invites more chronic diseases impacting your heart, brain, kidney and other vital organs.

Medications like beta-blockers blocks the action of hormones in the nervous system, such as epinephrine, also known as adrenaline. As a result, the nerve impulses traveling through the heart slows down. Hence, the heart rate slows down and pumps blood less forcefully around the body reducing your blood pressure. But, in a way the medicines are forcing your natural ability of heart pumping action making your heart weaker over the time.

Monitor your blood pressure regularly and try to avoid medicines if your blood pressure is elevated or you are pre-hypertensive. Elevated high blood pressure is a clear warning for you to change your lifestyle. Add physical activities and nutrition rich diet to your routine to achieve longevity and a healthier life.

Select an enjoyable form of exercise for yourself. This is about finding joy in movement and making time in your day that you look forward to, not just about "getting fit." Make sure it's something that speaks to your spirit, whether it's the stillness of yoga, the rhythm of dancing, cycling, running, or participating in a sport.

Make reasonable, attainable fitness objectives. Although heart health is the main purpose, setting more manageable, quantifiable goals can be highly motivating. It could be learning a new yoga pose, cutting a minute off your race, or walking an additional kilometer. Honor these accomplishments since they represent steps toward heart health.

A shorter workout is preferable than none at all on days when you are pressed for time or have poor energy. A quick ten-minute stroll counts toward your objective. Length is subordinated to consistency.

Take breaks when needed, adjust your workouts as needed, and consult a doctor if you have any health issues. Your workout regimen should honor the demands and constraints of your body. Exercise should be seen as a celebration of your body's abilities rather than an admission of guilt about what you eat.

Reach out to personal trainer and nutritionist to help you out with your training and nutrition plan if you have no idea and direction on how to start.

For those, who cannot afford the coaches as of now, my first two bestseller books on Amazon might help you in changing your lifestyle by adding fitness to your routine and helping you prepare your own nutrition plan by explaining the science behind the foods we choose.

Add Fitness to Lifestyle
https://www.amazon.com/Eat-Mindfully-Cheat-Wisely-Explaining/dp/B0CM9HTJ5X/

Eat Mindfully Cheat Wisely
https://www.amazon.com/Eat-Mindfully-Cheat-Wisely-Explaining/dp/B0CM9HTJ5X/

I know it seems like a promotion strategy for these two books, but for you, important is to just kick-start your journey towards a healthier life. So, choose whatever works with you, but please take your first step now and I assure that you won't regret!

All the best for your new active and healthy life!

Did this book help you in some way? If so, I would really appreciate your honest review so that it would help other people find the right book for their needs. This will also give me motivation to write more content and share more knowledge that I have.

Thank you in advance for sharing the review!

www.ingramcontent.com/pod-product-compliance
Lightning Source LLC
Chambersburg PA
CBHW070153230526
45471CB00002B/650